THE HEALING POWER OF SOMATIC THERAPY AND EXERCISES

The Ultimate Guide to Alleviating Stress, Pain, Anxiety, Trauma, and Daily Somatic Practices for Well-being

Kristi Tillson

Copyright@2024

TABLE OF CONTENTS

Chapter One

Introduction

In today's fast-paced world, stress, pain, anxiety, and trauma have become common experiences that impact millions of people worldwide. In today's fast-paced world, along with previous encounters and physical conditions, it is common to experience a disconnection between the mind and body. This disconnection can give rise to a range of mental and physical health concerns. Traditional therapeutic approaches have historically emphasized either mental or physical aspects, addressing symptoms separately. Nevertheless, an increasing amount of research and clinical experience indicates that taking a comprehensive approach, which considers both the psychological and physiological aspects, is essential for complete healing and overall wellness. Here is where somatic therapy comes into the picture.

Understanding Somatic Therapy

Somatic therapy is a comprehensive approach to healing that highlights the deep connection between the mind and body. The term "somatic" comes from the Greek word "soma," which translates to "body." Understanding the deep connection between the body and mind, somatic therapy recognizes the importance of physical sensations and bodily experiences in promoting emotional and psychological well-being. Unlike traditional talk therapies that primarily focus on cognitive and emotional processes, somatic therapy integrates body awareness, physical movement, and touch as essential elements of the healing process.

With a deep focus on bodily sensations, somatic therapy aims to enhance self-awareness and harness this newfound understanding to promote healing. It encompasses a range of methods aimed at enhancing individuals' body awareness, identifying physical signs of emotional concerns, and alleviating accumulated tension and trauma. These techniques encompass a variety of practices, including breathwork, mindfulness, Somatic Experiencing (SE), and Sensorimotor Psychotherapy.

The significance of addressing stress, anxiety, pain, and trauma

Addressing stress, anxiety, pain, and trauma is of utmost importance. These conditions have a significant impact on both quality of life and overall health and well-being. Chronic stress and anxiety can have a significant impact on your physical health, potentially leading to cardiovascular disease, weakened immune function, and gastrointestinal issues. When pain strikes, whether it's a temporary discomfort or a long-lasting condition, it can greatly hinder a person's daily activities and overall happiness. Unresolved trauma can have long-term impacts on both mental and physical well-being, leading to conditions like post-traumatic stress disorder (PTSD), depression, and chronic pain syndromes.

Stress is a natural response to perceived threats and challenges, activating the body's fight-or-flight mechanism. Although this response can be helpful during times of short-term, high-stress situations, long-term stress can cause the activation of this system to persist, leading to negative physiological changes. Chronic stress can cause anxiety, resulting in constant worry and fear that can disrupt daily life and cause physical symptoms like headaches, muscle tension, and fatigue.

Chronic pain can be a complex blend of physical and psychological sensations. Chronic pain often results in a sense of despair, sadness, and withdrawal from social interactions, which can create a difficult cycle to overcome.

Experiencing trauma can have long-lasting effects on both the mind and body. Physical pain, tension, or other somatic symptoms can be a result of traumatic experiences that get trapped in the body. Long after the traumatic event has occurred, the body retains a memory of the experience, resulting in continued emotional and physical discomfort.

With a deep understanding of the body-mind connection, somatic therapy offers a distinct and powerful method to tackle these concerns. Through a focus on bodily sensations and the connection between physical and psychological experiences, somatic therapy aids in the release of stored tension and trauma. This can lead to a reduction in stress, anxiety, pain, and symptoms associated with trauma.

The advantages of somatic therapy and exercises
There are numerous benefits to somatic therapy and exercises, going beyond just alleviating symptoms and instead fostering a sense of overall well-being and resilience. Through cultivating a stronger link between the mind and body, people can enhance their understanding of themselves, improve their ability to manage emotions, and achieve a greater sense of balance.

Developed Body Awareness: Somatic therapy assists individuals in becoming more in tune with their bodily sensations and signals. By being more aware of your body's signals, you can catch stress and tension early on and take action to prevent them from getting worse.

Emotional Regulation: Using techniques such as breathwork, mindfulness, and movement, somatic therapy helps individuals learn effective methods for regulating their emotions. Engaging in regular physical activity has been shown to have a positive impact on mental well-being. It can help alleviate feelings of anxiety, enhance mood, and strengthen resilience in the face of adversity.

Releasing Stored Trauma: Various forms of somatic therapy are specifically tailored to assist in the release of trauma that is stored in the body. Various techniques, like Somatic Experiencing (SE) and Sensorimotor Psychotherapy, can help individuals process and release traumatic memories, resulting in significant healing and recovery.

Pain Management: Chronic pain can be effectively

managed through the use of somatic exercises and therapies. Through understanding and addressing the emotional and psychological factors that contribute to pain, individuals can find relief and enhance their physical function.

Stress Reduction: Somatic practices like mindfulness meditation, progressive muscle relaxation, and grounding exercises can be incredibly effective in reducing stress. These practices are beneficial for calming the nervous system, promoting relaxation, and improving resilience to stress.

Enhanced Overall Well-being: Through the integration of mind and body, somatic therapy fosters a sense of holistic well-being. Regular practice of somatic techniques has been found to have numerous benefits, including improved physical health, emotional balance, and a greater sense of vitality and life satisfaction.

With a deep understanding of the mind-body connection, somatic therapy provides a holistic approach to healing and wellness. Through the integration of somatic exercises and techniques into everyday routines, people can effectively address and reduce stress, anxiety, pain, and trauma, resulting in improved overall well-being and quality of life. With the increasing recognition of the mind-body connection, somatic therapy emerges as a potent and life-changing approach that can effectively tackle the intricate and diverse aspects of human health and well-being.

Chapter Two
Exploring the World of Somatic Therapy

Somatic therapy is a powerful method of healing that recognizes the deep connection between the mind and body, leading to transformative results. Based on the understanding that our physical bodies are connected to our psychological experiences, somatic therapy combines different techniques to support overall well-being. This chapter explores the historical background, core principles, and different modalities of somatic therapy, offering a thorough overview of this powerful therapeutic approach.

A Brief Look into the Past

The origins of somatic therapy can be traced back to early 20th-century pioneers who embarked on a journey to investigate the intricate relationship between the body and mind. An influential figure in this field was Wilhelm Reich, an Austrian psychoanalyst and student of Sigmund Freud. Reich discussed the idea of "body armor," which pertains to the muscular tensions and contractions that arise from suppressed emotions and psychological defenses. He was confident that by relieving these tensions, individuals could tap into and address underlying emotional issues.

Reich's contributions formed the basis for the emergence of different somatic therapies. During the 1960s and 1970s, Alexander Lowen, a student of Reich, took these ideas to new heights with the establishment of Bioenergetic Analysis. This approach combines therapy techniques with physical exercises to assist individuals in releasing stored emotions and enhancing their bodily awareness.

Dr. Moshe Feldenkrais developed the Feldenkrais Method, a somatic education system that utilizes gentle movement and directed attention to enhance physical function and self-awareness. Another notable figure was Ida Rolf, the creator of Rolfing Structural Integration. Her innovative approach to bodywork focuses on realigning the body's structure to enhance function and provide relief from pain.

In the late 20th century, Somatic Experiencing (SE) emerged, thanks to the work of Dr. Peter Levine. Our approach focuses on resolving trauma by addressing the physiological responses stored in the body. Levine's work has made a significant impact on our understanding and treatment of trauma by focusing on the body's role in healing.

Key Principles of Somatic Therapy

Somatic therapy is based on a set of core principles that set it apart from traditional psychotherapeutic approaches:

Mind-Body Connection: The mind and body are interconnected, with each having a significant impact on the other. Somatic therapy acknowledges and explores this intricate connection. Emotions, thoughts, and physical sensations are viewed as interconnected elements of the human experience, and taking a holistic approach to addressing them can result in more effective healing.

Body Awareness and Mindfulness: Developing a strong sense of body awareness and mindfulness is a key aspect of somatic therapy. This approach focuses on fostering an understanding of bodily sensations and states. Practicing mindfulness can be beneficial for individuals looking to better connect with their physical experiences and gain insight into their emotional and psychological well-being.

Release of Stored Tension and Trauma: Somatic therapy suggests that emotional and psychological traumas can get trapped in the body, resulting in persistent tension and physical symptoms. Various techniques are employed to facilitate the release of these stored experiences, fostering healing and providing relief from symptoms.

Regulation of the Nervous System: Numerous therapies specialize in assisting individuals with the regulation of their autonomic nervous system, which is responsible for managing the body's stress response. By understanding how to soothe the nervous system, people can alleviate symptoms of anxiety, stress, and trauma.

Holistic Integration: Emphasizing the integration of the body, mind, and spirit, somatic therapy takes a holistic approach to healing. Healing is seen as a comprehensive process that takes into account all aspects of a person's experience.

Approaches in Somatic Therapy

There are various modalities within somatic therapy, each with its own set of techniques and areas of focus. Here are some of the most widely practised and recognized forms of somatic therapy:

Somatic Experiencing (SE): Somatic Experiencing (SE) developed by Dr. Peter Levine, is a therapy focused on trauma that aims to release the physical effects of trauma stored in the body. SE is founded on the principle that animals in their natural habitat naturally release the energy connected to traumatic experiences through physical shaking. Humans frequently suppress these innate reactions, resulting in the build-up of trauma within the body.

SE involves guiding individuals to gently revisit challenging memories and experiences while paying close attention to their bodily sensations. Through this process, people can gradually release the built-up energy linked to the trauma, resulting in a decrease in symptoms and a general feeling of relief.

Bioenergetic Analysis: Created by Alexander Lowen, Bioenergetic Analysis integrates psychotherapeutic techniques with physical exercises to assist individuals in releasing stored emotions and enhancing bodily awareness. This approach is rooted in the belief that emotional issues manifest in the body's posture, movement, and energy flow. Through a series of grounding techniques, focused breathing exercises, and expressive movements, individuals can effectively release tension and boost their vitality. Through a comprehensive approach that considers both the emotional and physical dimensions of an individual's well-being, Bioenergetic Analysis seeks to foster overall healing and personal development.

Feldenkrais Method: This method was developed by Dr. Moshe Feldenkrais. It is a system of somatic education that focuses on gentle movement and directed attention to enhance physical function and self-awareness. This approach recognizes the close relationship between the body and mind, emphasizing that enhancing physical movement can have a positive impact on overall well-being.

Experts in exercise and therapy help individuals by guiding them through a series of movements that aim to enhance their awareness of their usual movement patterns and discover more effective ways of moving. Through this process, individuals may experience enhanced posture, decreased discomfort, and heightened flexibility and coordination.

Rolfing Structural Integration: Ida Rolf, the mastermind behind Rolfing Structural Integration, created a remarkable bodywork technique that focuses on realigning the body's structure to enhance function and provide relief from pain. Practitioners of Rolfing utilize deep tissue manipulation techniques to alleviate tension and restore proper alignment of the body's connective tissues, also known as fascia. We aim to help you achieve a more balanced and aligned body, resulting in improved movement, reduced pain, and enhanced overall well-being. During Rolfing sessions, a series of treatments are used to gradually target various areas of the body and incorporate the resulting changes into the person's overall structure.

Sensorimotor Psychotherapy: Pat Ogden developed Sensorimotor Psychotherapy, which combines body-centred techniques with traditional talk therapy. This approach is highly beneficial in treating trauma and attachment issues, as it focuses on both the psychological and somatic aspects of these experiences.
Through the practice of Sensorimotor Psychotherapy, individuals are guided to develop a heightened awareness of their bodily sensations and movements. This process allows for a deeper exploration of how these physical experiences are interconnected with their emotional and psychological well-being. Through a comprehensive

approach that addresses both physical and mental well-being, this method strives to foster overall wellness and individual development.

Body-Mind Centering: Body-Mind Centering (BMC), created by Bonnie Bainbridge Cohen, offers a hands-on approach to exploring movement and consciousness. Our practitioners utilize movement, touch, and guided imagery to delve into the connections between the body, mind, and spirit.

BMC emphasizes the importance of understanding the body's internal processes and their impact on overall well-being. This approach can be highly effective in increasing self-awareness, enhancing physical function, and fostering emotional balance.

Exploring the Uses of Somatic Therapy

With its wide applicability to both physical and psychological issues, somatic therapy proves to be a versatile and effective approach to healing. Here are some of the main uses of somatic therapy:

Effective Stress and Anxiety Reduction Technique:

Somatic therapy techniques like breathwork, mindfulness,

and progressive muscle relaxation can help you regulate your nervous system and alleviate symptoms. Through a heightened sense of bodily awareness and a mindful approach to responding, individuals can cultivate a stronger ability to cope with stress and anxiety.

Trauma Healing: Somatic therapy is highly effective in treating trauma by focusing on the physiological responses stored in the body. Various techniques, like Somatic Experiencing and Sensorimotor Psychotherapy, can assist individuals in releasing the stored energy linked to trauma and incorporating the experience into their overall sense of self.

Pain Management: Chronic pain is often a complex experience that involves both physical and psychological aspects. Through somatic therapy, individuals can discover and let go of tension and stress that may be causing their pain. Methods like the Feldenkrais Method and Rolfing Structural Integration have been shown to enhance physical function and alleviate pain by targeting the root structural and movement patterns.

Emotional Regulation: Through heightened recognition of physical sensations and the practice of mindful responses, somatic therapy empowers individuals to cultivate improved emotional regulation abilities. Engaging in regular physical activity has the potential to enhance your mood, decrease emotional reactivity, and promote a greater sense of emotional equilibrium.

Enhanced Physical Function: Numerous somatic therapies prioritize the enhancement of physical movement and function. Discover powerful techniques that can improve flexibility, coordination, and overall physical health. These methods focus on addressing habitual movement patterns and increasing awareness of the body's internal processes.

Personal Growth and Self-Awareness: Somatic therapy facilitates a comprehensive understanding of oneself by integrating the physical, mental, and emotional aspects. Engaging in this practice can result in a deeper understanding of oneself, personal development, and a stronger bond with oneself and those around us.

Supporting Evidence for Somatic Therapy
There is a wealth of research that demonstrates the effectiveness of somatic therapy in addressing various physical and psychological concerns. Research has indicated that somatic therapies have been found to result in notable enhancements in symptoms related to anxiety, depression, PTSD, and chronic pain.
For instance, studies have shown that Somatic Experiencing can effectively alleviate symptoms of PTSD and stress related to trauma. A study published in the Journal of Traumatic Stress revealed that individuals who underwent SE experienced notable decreases in symptoms associated with PTSD when compared to a control group.

Similarly, research on the Feldenkrais Method has

demonstrated its ability to enhance physical function and alleviate pain in individuals with chronic pain conditions. A systematic review published in Evidence-Based Complementary and Alternative Medicine revealed that the Feldenkrais Method resulted in notable enhancements in pain management, mobility, and overall well-being for individuals dealing with chronic musculoskeletal pain. Studies have demonstrated that incorporating mindfulness-based somatic practices, like body scanning and mindful movement, can have beneficial impacts on mental well-being. A study published in Mindfulness revealed that engaging in body scanning meditation resulted in notable decreases in stress and anxiety levels among participants. These findings emphasize the effectiveness of somatic therapy in treating various physical and psychological concerns, making it a valuable contribution to the field of integrative medicine.

Appreciating the deep connection between the mind and body is key to understanding somatic therapy and the potential it holds for holistic healing. With a rich history dating back to the groundbreaking work of pioneers such as Wilhelm Reich and Alexander Lowen, somatic therapy has evolved into a versatile practice that can be applied to various areas such as trauma healing, stress reduction, and pain management.
The fundamental principles of somatic therapy focus on the connection between the mind and body, developing body awareness, releasing stored tension and trauma, regulating the nervous system, and achieving holistic integration. These principles offer a comprehensive approach to addressing both physical and psychological concerns. Through the integration of somatic therapy, individuals can enhance their self-awareness, regulate their emotions, and improve their overall well-being.
With the ever-changing landscape of the field and the

growing body of research backing its effectiveness, somatic therapy emerges as a powerful and holistic method for promoting overall well-being. Utilized as a standalone treatment or in combination with other therapeutic methods, somatic therapy provides a pathway to profound healing and a greater sense of unity between the mind and body.

Chapter Three

Effective Techniques for Stress Relief through Somatic Exercises

Stress is a common aspect of life, but when it becomes a constant presence, it can have a significant impact on our overall well-being, affecting both our physical and mental health. Discover the incredible benefits of somatic exercises, which provide a comprehensive method for effectively managing stress. By focusing on the connection between the mind and body, these exercises promote relaxation and enhance self-awareness. These exercises utilize a range of techniques to help individuals develop a greater awareness of their bodily sensations, alleviate physical tension, and foster a state of tranquility and overall wellness. In this chapter, we will delve into a variety of somatic exercises that are specifically tailored to help alleviate stress. These exercises include breathwork techniques, progressive muscle relaxation, grounding exercises, and more.

Breathwork Techniques

Understanding the importance of proper breathing goes beyond its basic function in sustaining life. It has a significant influence on both our physical and mental well-being. Being mindful of your breath and practicing controlled breathing techniques can activate the parasympathetic nervous system, leading to a sense of relaxation and a decrease in stress levels. There are various breathwork techniques that can help reduce stress:

Diaphragmatic or Belly Breathing: Engage the diaphragm fully while breathing for optimal results. This method is effective in enhancing oxygen intake and inducing a state of relaxation.

Here is how to practice:
- Find a position that feels comfortable, whether sitting or lying down.
- Position one hand on your chest and the other on your abdomen.
- Breathe in deeply through your nose, allowing your abdomen to rise while keeping your chest relatively still.
- Breathe out slowly through your mouth or nose, noticing your abdomen sinking.
- Continue the exercise for a few minutes, directing your attention to the expansion and contraction of your abdomen.

Box Breathing: This technique, also referred to as square breathing, incorporates a sequence of inhaling, holding the breath, exhaling, and holding the breath once more, all for a count of four. It is frequently utilized by individuals in high-performance fields to alleviate stress and improve focus.

Here's a simple way to practice:
- Find a comfortable position and make sure your back is straight.
- Breathe in slowly through your nose for a count of four.
- Take a deep breath and hold it for a count of four.
- Breathe out slowly through your mouth, counting to four.
- Take a deep breath and hold it for a count of four.
- Continue the cycle for a few minutes.

Alternate Nostril Breathing: This is a yogic practice called NadiShodhana that promotes a balanced nervous system and a calm mind.

Here's a simple way to practice:
- Find a comfortable seated position with your back straight.
- Using your right thumb, gently close your right nostril and take a deep breath in through your left nostril.
- Use your ring finger to close your left nostril, then release your thumb and exhale through your right nostril.
- Breathe in through your right nostril, then use your thumb to close it.
- Let go of your ring finger and breathe out through your left nostril.
- Keep switching between nostrils for a few minutes, paying attention to your breath.

Progressive Muscle Relaxation: This is a technique that can help you relax your muscles and reduce stress. It involves tensing and then releasing different muscle groups in your body. By practicing this technique regularly, you can learn to recognize and release tension in your muscles, promoting a sense of calm and relaxation.

Progressive muscle relaxation (PMR) is a method that focuses on tensing and then releasing various muscle groups in the body. This approach is effective in alleviating physical tension and fostering a sense of relaxation. PMR can be highly beneficial for individuals who struggle with muscle tightness caused by stress.

How to Practice

- Discover a serene and cozy spot to settle in.
- Take a moment to close your eyes and focus on your breath.
- Beginning with your feet, contract the muscles as tightly as you can for approximately five seconds.
- Let go of the tension suddenly and experience the sensation of deep relaxation.
- Move to the next muscle group (such as calves, thighs, abdomen, arms, shoulders, face) and repeat the sequence.
- Work your way the whole body focusing on each muscle group individually.
- Once you finish the sequence, take a moment to savor the feeling of relaxation throughout your entire body.

Grounding Techniques

Grounding exercises are specifically crafted to assist individuals in establishing a strong connection with the present moment and their immediate surroundings. These techniques are highly effective in reducing stress and anxiety by redirecting attention away from worry and towards the present moment.

5-4-3-2-1 Technique: This grounding exercise utilizes the five senses to focus on the present moment.

Here's a simple practice:
- Find a comfortable seated position and take a few deep breaths.
- Take a moment to observe your surroundings and identify five things that catch your attention.
- Identify four things that you can touch or feel.
- Take a moment to listen and identify three sounds around you.
- Identify two scents that you can detect
- Think of one thing you can taste.
- Pause for a moment and reflect on how you feel after completing the exercise.

Body Scan: This mindful practice focuses on paying attention various parts of the body, observing sensations, and letting go of any tension.

Here's a simple way to practice:
- Find a comfortable position, either lying down or sitting, and gently close your eyes.
- Take a moment to breathe deeply and find a sense of relaxation.

- Direct your attention towards your toes and become aware of any sensations you may feel.
- Gradually shift your focus from your feet to your legs, then move up to your abdomen, chest, arms, neck, and face.
- Take note of each area as you go through the various parts of the body.
- If you happen to feel any tension, simply take a deep breath and visualize releasingit.
- Continue until you've scanned your entire body.

Grounding Through Movement: Embracing mindful movement can provide a sense of grounding in the present moment and alleviate stress. Various practices like yoga, Tai Chi, or simply going for a mindful walk can be beneficial.

How to practice:
- Choose a type of movement that you genuinely enjoy and can do with full mindfulness.
- Pay close attention to the physical sensations you experience while you engage in movement.
- Pay close attention to the sensations in your muscles, the way your body moves, and the synchronization of your breath with your movements.

- When your mind starts to drift, gently redirect your attention to the physical sensations.

Somatic Movement Practices.
Integrating physical activity such as movement into your daily routine can greatly reduce stress levels and promote a sense of relaxation for both your body and mind. Engage in somatic movement practices to experience the benefits of gentle, mindful movements that promote body awareness and alleviate tension.

Gentle Yoga: This practice integrates gentle physical movements, controlled breathing techniques, and mindfulness to enhance relaxation and alleviate stress. Practicing gentle yoga, like Hatha or Restorative yoga, can be highly beneficial for reducing stress.

How to Practice
- Creating a suitable environment is essential for effective practice. Locate a calm and uninterrupted space where you can fully focus on your practice.
- Start by dedicating a few moments to deep breathing, allowing yourself to find inner balance.
- Engage in a sequence of gentle poses, directing your attention to your breath and the physical sensations you experience.
- Incoperate poses that encourage relaxation, like Child's Pose, Cat-Cow, and Legs-Up-The-Wall.

- Conclude your practice by dedicating a few minutes to Savasana (Corpse Pose) in order to achieve complete relaxation and allow the benefits to fully sink in.

Tai Chi: This is a practice that incorporates slow, flowing movements and deep breathing techniques. It is beneficial activity that can help reduce stress and enhance overall well-being.

Here is a Simple way to Practice

- Finding a quiet environment for your practice is essential. Look for a calm and peaceful space where you can fully concentrate without distractions.
- Start by dedicating a few minutes to deep breathing in order to center yourself.
- Learn Tai Chi sequence by following the guidance of a knowledgeable instructor or instructional video.
- Take your time as you go through the sequence, slowly, mindfully and attentive to each movement and your breathing.
- Make sure to consistently engage in Tai Chi to fully reap its long-term benefits.

Qigong is a practice that incorporates gentle movements, breath control, and meditation to enhance energy flow and alleviate stress.

How to Practice
- Creating a suitable environment for your practice is essential. Look for a

calm and peaceful space where you
can fully focus without distractions.

- Start by dedicating a few moments to deep breathing to center yourself.
- Discover the basic Qigong sequence by following the guidance of a knowledgeable instructor or instructional video.
- Take your time as you go through the sequence, slowly, mindfully and aware of your breath and the way your body feels.
- Practice regularly to reap the rewards of Qigong.

Mindfulness Meditation

This is incredibly beneficial for your overall well-being. Practicing mindfulness meditation entails directing your attention to the present moment with a non-judgmental attitude. Engaging in this practice can have a positive impact on your well-being by fostering a sense of calm and enhancing your self-awareness.

Here's how to practice:

- Locate a peaceful and cozy spot to either sit or lie down.
- Take a moment to close your eyes and take a few deep breaths.
- Direct your focus towards your breath, observing the feeling of the air flowing in and out of your body.
- When your mind starts to wander, simply redirect your attention back to your breath without any self-criticism.

- Keep going for a few minutes, slowly extending the time as you get more at ease with the practice.

Visualization Techniques

Visualization entails harnessing the power of your imagination to calming and positive image. This technique is effective in reducing stress as it promotes relaxation and a sense of peace.

Here is how to practice:

- Find a serene and cozy spot to either sit or lie down.
- Take a moment to close your eyes and focus on your breath.
- Picture yourself in a peaceful and calming scene, like a beautiful beach, lush forest, or majestic mountain.
- Engage all of your senses to create a vivid scene, immersing yourself in the sights, sounds, smells, and sensations.
- Take a moment to immerse yourself in the scene, allowing your mind to unwind and savor the moment.

Self-Massage Techniques

Self-massage is beneficial for relieving physical tension and inducing a state of relaxation. Various techniques, including acupressure and gentle muscle kneading, can be highly effective in providing relief from stress.

Here's how to practice:

- Locate a quiet and cozy spot to either sit or lie down.
- Apply gentle pressure to areas of tension, such as your shoulders, neck, and temples using your fingers.
- Employ circular motions to gently massage the muscles, paying special attention to areas that may be experiencing tightness or discomfort.
- Take a few moments to gently massage each area, allowing yourself to breathe deeply and fully immerse in the soothing sensation of relaxation.

Journaling and somatic writing

Journaling is a beneficial method of working through emotions and managing stress. When you engage in somatic writing, you direct your attention to the physical sensations within your body while expressing your experiences and emotions through writing.

How to Practice:
- Find a quiet and cozy spot to settle down with a journal and pen.
- Take a moment to focus and breathe deeply.
- Start documenting your present experiences and emotions, while being mindful of any physical sensations that may arise during the writing process.

- Pay attention to the sensations in your body as you write down your thoughts and emotions.
- Keep writing for as long as you feel at ease, using this process to let go of tension and gain a better understanding of what causes you stress.

Incorporating Somatic Exercises into Your Daily Routine

Integrating somatic exercises into your daily routine can be a valuable tool for effectively managing stress and enhancing your overall well-being. Here is a sample daily routine that incorporates a range of somatic techniques:

My Morning Routine:

- Begin your day by dedicating a few minutes to diaphragmatic breathing, allowing yourself to find inner balance.
- Participate in a brief session of gentle yoga or Tai Chi to invigorate your body and mind.

Midday Break:
- Take a few moments to engage in the 5-4-3-2-1 grounding technique to

regain focus and alleviate stress.

- Take a few moments to engage in mindful breathing or a body scan to help alleviate any tension you may be feeling.

Evening Routine:
- Learn a technique called progressive muscle relaxation to help you relax and get a good night's sleep.
- Try a visualization technique before going to sleep to help you relax and find inner peace.

During the day:
- Integrate mindful moments into your routine, like deep breathing, self-massage, or journaling, to effectively handle stress as it comes up.
- Utilize grounding techniques when faced with stressful situations to maintain a sense of presence and tranquility.
Discover the power of somatic exercises, a holistic approach that tackles stress by bridging the mind and body. Practicing various techniques like breathwork, progressive muscle relaxation, grounding exercises, and mindful movement can assist individuals in becoming more aware of their bodily sensations, relieving physical tension, and fostering a sense of calm and well-being. Through the integration of these exercises into a daily regimen, individuals can

develop a greater ability to cope with stress and improve their overall well-being. Whether practiced individually or in combination, somatic exercises offer valuable techniques for achieving and maintaining stress relief and overall well-being.

Chapter Four

Exploring Somatic Approaches for Anxiety Management

Anxiety is a widespread and frequently incapacitating condition that impacts countless individuals across the globe. Although cognitive-behavioral therapy (CBT) and medication are commonly used and proven effective, somatic approaches provide distinct and potent techniques for anxiety management by focusing on the connection between the mind and body. These methods emphasize the connection between physical sensations, bodily movements, and awareness, and how they can impact emotional states and vice versa. In this section, we will delve into a range of somatic techniques that can help you effectively manage anxiety. These techniques include grounding exercises, body awareness practices, breathwork, movement therapies, and more.

Gaining insight into the physical origins of anxiety

Before delving into specific somatic techniques, it's crucial to grasp the ways in which anxiety presents itself in the body. When anxiety strikes, our bodies can go into a fight-or-flight mode as a natural response to what we perceive as threats. This response involves the activation of the body's sympathetic nervous system, resulting in symptoms like a higher heart rate, shallow breathing, tense muscles, and a feeling of restlessness. By directly addressing these physical symptoms, somatic approaches can effectively interrupt the anxiety cycle and encourage a state of calm.

Grounding Exercises

Grounding exercises are techniques that assist individuals in connecting with the present moment and their physical bodies, offering a sense of stability and calmness. These exercises are highly effective in managing anxiety, as they redirect attention away from anxious thoughts and towards physical sensations.

5-4-3-2-1 Technique: This sensory awareness exercise utilizes the five senses to focus on the present moment. **Here's a simple way to practice:**

- Find a comfortable seated position and take a few deep breaths.
- Take a moment to observe your surroundings and identify five things that catch your attention
- Identify four things that you can touch or feel.
- Identify three sounds around you or that you can hear.
- Identify two things that scent around you.
- Identify one thing you can taste.

- Take a moment to reflect on how you feel after you've finished the exercise.

Grounding with the Earth

Connecting physically with the ground can provide a powerful sense of stability and calm.

Here's how to practice:

- Locate a peaceful outdoor area where you can comfortably sit or stand without shoes on.
- Take a moment to close your eyes and take a deep breath.
- Feel the tactile connection with the earth beneath your feet.
- Imagine a strong connectionbetween your feet and the ground,or roots growing from your feet into the ground, holding you firmly.
- Take a moment to reflect on the connection between your body and the earth.

Body Scan Meditation: This mindfulness practice focuses on bringing awareness to various areas of the body, observing the sensations present, and letting go of any tension that may be present.

Here's a simple way to practice:

- Find a comfortable position, either lying down or sitting, and gently close your eyes.
- Take a deep breath to find a sense of relaxation.
- Direct your attention towards your toes and become aware of any sensations you may feel.
- Gradually shift your focus from your feet to your legs, then move up to your abdomen, chest, arms, neck, and face. Take the time to be mindful of each area as you go.

- If you happen to sense any tension, simply take a deep breath and envision letting it go.
- Continue until you have scanned your entire body.

Body Awareness Practices

Engaging in body awareness practices can assist individuals to develop a deeper connections with their bodily sensations and gaining insight into the ways these sensations intertwine with their emotions. Through a heightened sense of body awareness, individuals are able to more effectively recognize and address the physical manifestations of anxiety.

Focusing Technique: Eugene Gendlin developed a method that involves directing your attention to the internal awareness of a situation or feeling, known as the "felt sense" of the body.

Here's how to practice:

- Find a peaceful spot where you can sit comfortably.
- Take a moment to close your eyes and take a deep breath.
- Direct your focus to the core of your body, specifically the area encompassing your chest and abdomen.
- Pay attention to any physical sensations or feelings that you experience.
- Embrace the sensation, explore it without any judgment or the urge to alter it.
- Take a moment to pause and reflect on any new insights or changes in your feelings.

Somatic Tracking: Engaging in somatic tracking involves attentively observing physical sensations with a sense of curiosity and openness, refraining from any form of judgment.

Here's how to practice:
- Find a comfortable position, either sitting or lying down.
- Take a moment to close your eyes and take a deep breath.
- Direct your attention to a particular region of your body where you experience anxiety, like your chest or stomach.
- Pay attention to the sensations in that area, and make a mental note of their intensity, shape, and movement.
- Stay with the sensation and let it change naturally.
- Reflect on any change in your emotional well-being after the exercise.

Interceptive Awareness: Developing interoceptive awareness entails focusing on internal bodily sensations, including heartbeat, breath, and muscle tension.

Here's a simple practice you can try:

- Find a comfortable seated position and gently close your eyes.
- Remember to take a few deep breaths and center your attention on your internal sensations.
  Pay attention to your heartbeat, the rhythm of your breath, and any tightness in your muscles.
  Take a moment to observe these sensations without passing any judgment, just simply notice them.

Keep going for a few minutes, staying mindful of your internal sensations.

Deep breathing techniques

Mastering breathwork techniques is essential for effectively managing anxiety through somatic approaches. Being mindful of your breath and practicing controlled breathing techniques can have a positive impact on your overall well-being. It can help bring balance to your autonomic nervous system, alleviate stress, and induce a state of relaxation.

Diaphragmatic Breathing: This technique involves engaging the diaphragm to promote relaxation.

Here's a simple way to practice: Find a comfortable position, either sitting or lying down.
Position one hand on your chest and the other on your abdomen.
Breathe in deeply through your nose, allowing your abdomen to rise while keeping your chest relatively still.
Breathe out slowly through your mouth or nose, noticing your abdomen sinking.
Continue the exercise for a few minutes, directing your attention to the gentle expansion and contraction of your abdomen.
Box Breathing: This technique requires inhaling, holding the breath, exhaling, and holding the breath again, each for a count of four.

Here's a simple way to practice: Find a comfortable position and make sure your back is straight.
Breathe in slowly through your nose for a count of four.
Take a deep breath and hold it for a count of four.

Breathe out slowly through your mouth, counting to four.
Take a deep breath and hold it for a count of four.
Continue the cycle for a few minutes.
Alternate Nostril Breathing is a yogic practice called NadiShodhana that promotes a balanced nervous system and a calm mind.

Here's a simple way to practice: Find a comfortable seated position with your spine aligned.
Place your right thumb over your right nostril and take a deep breath in through your left nostril.
Use your ring finger to close your left nostril, then release your thumb and exhale through your right nostril.
Breathe in through your right nostril, then use your thumb to close it.
Let go of your ring finger and breathe out through your left nostril.
Keep switching between nostrils for a few minutes, paying attention to your breathing.
Expert in movement therapies
Physical movement is utilized in movement therapies to help alleviate tension, enhance body awareness, and diminish anxiety. There is a wide variety of therapies available, ranging from structured practices like yoga and Tai Chi to more spontaneous forms of movement.

Yoga is a practice that incorporates various physical postures, breath control, and meditation techniques to help promote relaxation and alleviate feelings of anxiety.

Creating a suitable environment for your practice is essential. Look for a peaceful area where you can focus without any disturbances.

Start by dedicating a few moments to deep breathing, allowing yourself to find a sense of inner calm and focus.

Engage in a sequence of soothing poses, directing your attention to your breath and the physical sensations you experience.

Include poses that encourage relaxation, like Child's Pose, Cat-Cow, and Legs-Up-The-Wall.

Conclude your practice by dedicating a few minutes to Savasana (Corpse Pose) for complete relaxation and to fully absorb the positive effects.

Tai Chi is a practice that incorporates gentle, fluid movements and focused breathing. Many people find this activity to be a calming and beneficial practice, helping to alleviate stress and enhance their overall state of mind.

Creating a suitable environment for your practice is essential. Look for a calm and peaceful area where you can fully concentrate without any interruptions.

Start by dedicating a few moments to deep breathing, allowing yourself to find a sense of calm and focus.

Discover the art of Tai Chi by following the guidance of a knowledgeable instructor or instructional video.

Take your time and be fully present as you go through each movement, paying attention to the way your body moves and your breath.

Consistent practice is key to fully reap the rewards of Tai Chi.

Qigong is a practice that incorporates gentle movements, breath control, and meditation to enhance energy flow and alleviate feelings of anxiety.

Creating a suitable environment for practice is essential. Look for a calm and peaceful space where you can fully focus and avoid any potential distractions.
Start by dedicating a few moments to deep breathing, allowing yourself to find a sense of calm and focus.
Discover the fundamentals of Qigong by following the guidance of a knowledgeable instructor or instructional video.
Take your time as you go through the sequence, paying close attention to your breath and the way your body feels.
Consistency is key when it comes to reaping the rewards of Qigong.
Dance/Movement Therapy: This therapeutic approach utilizes the power of expressive movement to address emotional, cognitive, and physical concerns. It can have a significant impact on reducing anxiety and enhancing mood.

Here's how you can practice: Locate a suitable area where you have ample room to move around without any disturbances.
Choose music that speaks to you and motivates you to get moving.
Embrace the freedom of allowing your body to naturally respond to the music, tuning into the sensations and emotions that arise.
Release any preconceived notions or assumptions about your movements and savor the experience.
Take a moment to consider your emotions and any valuable insights you may have gained from your workout.
Incorporating Somatic Approaches into Everyday

Activities

Integrating somatic practices into your daily routines can be a valuable tool for effectively managing anxiety and enhancing your overall well-being. Here are some practical tips for incorporating these techniques into your daily routine:

My Morning Routine:
Begin your day by dedicating a few minutes to diaphragmatic breathing, allowing yourself to find inner balance.
Participate in a brief yoga or Tai Chi session to invigorate your body and mind.

Take a midday break:
Spend a few moments engaging in the 5-4-3-2-1 grounding technique to regain focus and alleviate feelings of anxiety.
Take a few moments to engage in mindful breathing or a body scan to help release any tension you may be experiencing.

Evening Routine:
Try incorporating progressive muscle relaxation or a body scan into your routine to help you unwind from the day and get ready for a peaceful night's sleep.
Try incorporating a visualization technique into your bedtime routine for a more relaxed and peaceful state of mind.

During the course of the day:
Integrate moments of mindfulness into your routine, like deep breathing, self-massage, or spontaneous movement, to effectively handle anxiety as it comes up.
Utilize grounding techniques when faced with

stressful situations to maintain a sense of presence and tranquility.

Utilizing somatic approaches to manage anxiety can provide individuals with powerful tools to address the mind-body connection, resulting in relief from anxiety symptoms and an overall improvement in well-being. Various techniques, including grounding exercises, body awareness practices, breathwork, and movement therapies, can assist individuals in developing a greater awareness of their physical sensations, alleviating tension, and fostering a state of tranquility. Through the incorporation of these practices into everyday activities, individuals can develop a stronger ability to cope with anxiety and improve their overall well-being. Utilizing somatic approaches can be incredibly beneficial for effectively managing anxiety in a holistic and integrative manner, whether used individually or in combination.

Chapter Five
Effective Techniques for Managing Pain

Chronic pain is a widespread issue that impacts countless individuals globally, often resulting in considerable physical, emotional, and psychological suffering. Conventional methods of managing pain, like medication and physical therapy, can be effective, but they may not fully address the complex nature of chronic pain. An integrative approach to pain management is offered through somatic techniques, which emphasize the mind-body connection. This approach focuses on body awareness, movement, breath, and mindfulness. These techniques are effective in helping individuals alleviate pain, enhance their overall function, and improve their quality of life.

Exploring the Somatic Approach to Pain
Understanding the close connection between the mind and body is fundamental to somatic pain management techniques. Understanding pain goes beyond the physical realm and encompasses emotional and psychological aspects as well. By taking a comprehensive approach to these components, somatic techniques can effectively

manage pain perception and enhance coping strategies. Important components of the somatic approach are:

Developing a heightened sense of bodily sensations and movements to recognize and alleviate tension or stress. Discover the power of breathwork, a practice that harnesses controlled breathing techniques to help regulate the nervous system and alleviate stress caused by pain. Practicing mindfulness and meditation can help cultivate present-moment awareness, allowing you to shift your focus away from pain and reduce emotional distress. Discover the power of gentle, mindful movement to enhance your mobility, flexibility, and ability to manage pain.
Practices for Enhancing Body Awareness
Practicing body awareness can enhance one's ability to recognize and alleviate physical discomfort and tension. These practices typically incorporate a focus on being present and incorporating gentle movements.

Body Scan Meditation: This technique encourages individuals to mindfully scan their bodies, paying attention to any areas that may be experiencing tension or discomfort.

Here's how to practice: Locate a peaceful and cozy spot to either lie down or sit.

Take a moment to close your eyes and focus on your breath.

Start by directing your attention to your toes and becoming aware of any sensations you may feel, whether it's tension or relaxation.

Gradually shift your focus from your feet to your legs, then up to your hips, abdomen, chest, arms, neck, and face. Take note of any sensations you experience without forming any judgments.

When you come across areas of tension or pain, try taking deep breaths and visualizing the release of that tension with each exhale.

Keep scanning until you reach the top of your head.

Centering: Created by Eugene Gendlin, focusing entails directing your attention to the sensations in your body that are connected to pain or discomfort.

Here's a simple way to practice: Find a comfortable spot and gently close your eyes.
Take a moment to focus and breathe deeply.
Focus your attention on the specific area of your body that is causing you pain or discomfort.
Take a moment to simply observe the sensation, paying attention to its characteristics such as size, shape, texture, and movement.
Embrace the sensation, accepting it without any negative

thoughts or pushback.

Take a moment to consider any new understandings or changes in how you view the pain.

Discover the transformative power of Somatic Experiencing, a technique pioneered by Peter Levine. This approach targets the release of stored trauma in the body, offering relief from pain and tension.

Here's how to practice: Find a position that feels comfortable, whether sitting or lying down.

Take a moment to breathe deeply and find a sense of relaxation.

Direct your focus to the specific area of your body that is causing you pain or discomfort.

Pay attention to any sensations, emotions, or images that come up.

Embrace and fully immerse yourself in these sensations, without attempting to alter them.

Over time, as you continue to focus on the sensations, pay attention to any shifts or alterations in your experience.

Exploring Breathwork Techniques

Understanding and practicing breathwork techniques can have a profound impact on how we perceive pain. By regulating the autonomic nervous system and promoting relaxation, these techniques can make a significant difference. Practicing mindful and regulated breathing can be beneficial in managing stress and anxiety, especially when dealing with chronic pain.

Diaphragmatic Breathing: This technique involves engaging the diaphragm to promote relaxation and reduce pain.

Here's a simple way to practice: Find a comfortable sitting or lying position.

Position one hand on your chest and the other on your abdomen.

Breathe in deeply through your nose, allowing your belly to expand while keeping your chest steady.

Breathe out slowly through your mouth or nose, noticing your abdomen sinking.

Continue the exercise for a few minutes, paying attention to the expansion and contraction of your abdomen.

Box Breathing: This technique requires inhaling, holding the breath, exhaling, and holding the breath again, each for a count of four.

Here's a simple way to practice: Find a comfortable position and make sure your back is straight.

Breathe in slowly through your nose for a count of four.

Take a deep breath and hold it for a count of four.

Breathe out slowly through your mouth, counting to four.

Take a deep breath and hold it for a count of four.

Continue the cycle for a few minutes.

Alternate Nostril Breathing is a yogic practice called NadiShodhana that promotes a balanced nervous system and a calm mind.

Tips for Practicing:

Find a comfortable seated position with good posture.

Using your right thumb, gently close your right nostril and take a deep breath in through your left nostril.

Use your ring finger to close your left nostril, then release your thumb and exhale through your right nostril.

Breathe in through your right nostril, then use your thumb to close it.

Let go of your ring finger and breathe out through your left nostril.

Keep switching between nostrils for a few minutes, placing your attention on your breath.

Practicing mindfulness and meditation
Practicing mindfulness and meditation involves directing
your attention to the present moment without passing
judgment. These techniques can assist in redirecting focus
from discomfort and alleviating the emotional strain linked
to persistent pain.
Practicing mindfulness meditation can be beneficial for
reducing pain and stress by focusing on the present moment
without judgment.

Here's how to practice: Locate a peaceful and cozy spot to
either sit or lie down.
Take a moment to close your eyes and focus on your
breath.
Direct your focus towards your breath, observing the
feeling of the air as it flows in and out of your body.
If your mind starts to drift towards feelings of discomfort,
gently redirect your attention back to your breath.
Keep going for a few minutes, slowly extending the time as
you get more at ease with the routine.

Practicing Loving-Kindness Meditation: This meditation
practice emphasizes the development of empathy and
goodwill towards oneself and others, which can be
beneficial in alleviating emotional distress associated with
pain.
Here's a simple way to practice: Find a comfortable
seated position and gently close your eyes.
Take a moment to breathe deeply and find relaxation.
Quietly recite affirmations like "May I experience
happiness, may I enjoy good health, may I be free from
discomfort."
Spread these well-wishes to others, using phrases like "May
you experience happiness, may you enjoy good health, may
you be free from suffering."

Keep going for a few minutes, directing your attention towards the emotions of empathy and benevolence.

Guided Imagery: This technique utilizes the power of mental images to foster a state of tranquility and ease, ultimately aiding in the alleviation of pain.

Here's how to practice: Locate a peaceful and cozy spot to either sit or lie down.

Take a moment to close your eyes and focus on your breath.

Visualize a serene and tranquil setting, like a beach, forest, or mountain.

Engage all of your senses to create a vibrant scene, immersing yourself in the sights, sounds, smells, and sensations.

Take a few moments to immerse yourself in the scene, allowing your mind to fully unwind and savor the moment.

Expert in the field of movement therapy

Physical movement is utilized in movement therapies to alleviate tension, enhance mobility, and alleviate pain.

Various therapies can incorporate structured practices such as yoga and Tai Chi, along with more spontaneous forms of movement.

Yoga is a wonderful practice that combines physical postures, breath control, and meditation to help you relax and alleviate pain.

Creating a suitable environment for your practice is essential. Locate a calm and uninterrupted space where you can fully focus.

Start by dedicating a few moments to deep breathing, allowing yourself to find a sense of calm and focus.

Engage in a sequence of soothing poses, directing your attention to your breath and the physical sensations you experience.

Include poses that encourage relaxation and alleviate pain,

like Child's Pose, Cat-Cow, and Legs-Up-The-Wall. Conclude your practice by taking a few moments to rest in Savasana (Corpse Pose) and allow yourself to fully relax and absorb the benefits.

Tai Chi is a practice that incorporates gentle, fluid movements and focused breathing techniques. Many people find this activity to be a form of moving meditation that can help alleviate pain and enhance their overall sense of well-being.
Creating a suitable environment for your practice is essential. Look for a calm and peaceful area where you can fully focus without any interruptions.
Start by dedicating a few moments to deep breathing, allowing yourself to find a sense of calm and focus.
Discover the art of Tai Chi by following the guidance of a skilled instructor or instructional video.
Take your time as you go through the sequence, paying close attention to each movement and your breathing. Consistent practice is key to fully reap the rewards of Tai Chi.

Qigong: A practice that incorporates gentle movements, breath control, and meditation to enhance energy flow and alleviate discomfort.
Creating a suitable environment for your practice is essential. Look for a calm and peaceful space where you can fully focus without any interruptions.
Start by dedicating a few moments to deep breathing in order to find your inner balance.
Discover the fundamentals of Qigong by following the guidance of a knowledgeable instructor or instructional video.
Take your time as you go through the sequence, being fully present and aware of your breath and the way your body feels.

Consistency is key when it comes to reaping the rewards of Qigong. Make it a habit to practice regularly and you'll start to see the positive effects build up over time.

Dance/Movement Therapy: This therapeutic approach utilizes the power of expressive movement to effectively address emotional, cognitive, and physical concerns. It has shown great effectiveness in alleviating pain and enhancing mood.

Here's how you can practice: Locate a suitable area where you have ample room to move around without any disturbances.

Choose music that speaks to you and motivates you to get moving.

Embrace the freedom of allowing your body to naturally respond to the music, tuning into the sensations and emotions that arise.

Release any preconceived notions or demands regarding your physical actions and savor the moment.

Take a moment to consider your emotions and any valuable realizations that may have come to light during your workout.

Discover the power of incorporating somatic techniques into your everyday routine.

Integrating somatic practices into your daily routines can be a valuable tool for effectively managing pain and enhancing your overall well-being. Here are some practical tips for incorporating these strategies into your daily routine:

Start your day off right with a refreshing morning routine:

Begin your day by dedicating a few moments to diaphragmatic breathing, allowing yourself to find inner balance.

Participate in a brief session of yoga or Tai Chi to

invigorate your body and mind.

Take a midday break:

Take a few minutes to engage in a body scan or focusing technique to identify and release tension.

Take a few moments to engage in mindful breathing or guided imagery, which can help alleviate pain and reduce stress.

Evening Routine:

Try incorporating progressive muscle relaxation or a body scan into your routine to help you unwind from the day and get ready for a peaceful night's sleep.

Try incorporating a visualization technique into your bedtime routine for a more peaceful and relaxed state of mind.

During the course of the day:

Integrate mindful moments into your routine to effectively manage pain as it comes up. This can include taking deep breaths, practicing self-massage, or engaging in spontaneous movement.

Utilize grounding techniques in moments of stress to maintain a sense of presence and tranquility.

Utilizing somatic techniques for pain management provides a comprehensive approach that acknowledges the connection between the mind and body, resulting in pain relief and improved overall well-being. Practices like body awareness, breathwork, mindfulness, and movement therapies can assist individuals in becoming more in tune with their physical sensations, reducing tension, and fostering a sense of calm. Through the incorporation of these techniques into everyday activities, people can develop a stronger ability to cope with pain and enhance their overall well-being. Whether used individually or in combination, somatic approaches offer valuable and effective strategies for pain management in a holistic and integrative manner.

Chapter Six

Discover the power of somatic practices in healing trauma.

Experiencing trauma can have profound and enduring effects on both the mind and body. Conventional therapeutic methods, like talk therapy, typically prioritize the cognitive and emotional aspects of trauma, but may not fully address the physical effects that trauma has on the body. Utilizing somatic practices can provide effective tools for healing trauma by directly addressing bodily sensations and movements, emphasizing the mind-body connection. These practices are beneficial for individuals to release stored trauma in the body, regain a sense of safety, and develop resilience.

Exploring the Connection Between Trauma and the Body Understanding trauma involves recognizing it as a deeply distressing experience that overwhelms a person's ability to cope, resulting in feelings of helplessness and a disturbance in the body's equilibrium. Various traumatic experiences can encompass instances of physical or emotional abuse, accidents, natural disasters, and other life-threatening events. After experiencing trauma, individuals may develop a variety of symptoms such as anxiety, depression, hypervigilance, dissociation, and chronic pain.

Understanding the body's role in trauma is crucial. When faced with a traumatic event, the body instinctively enters a state of fight, flight, or freeze, which is controlled by the autonomic nervous system. Physiological imprints, such as tension, pain, and altered breathing patterns, can persist long after the traumatic event has ended. Somatic practices focus on addressing these imprints by helping individuals release stored trauma and fostering self-regulation and healing.

Somatic practices are essential for healing trauma. Somatic Experiencing (SE) is a powerful approach that can help individuals heal and recover from past traumas. It focuses on the connection between the mind and body, allowing for a deeper understanding and release of stored tension and stress. Through gentle and mindful exercises, SE can guide individuals towards a greater sense of well-being and resilience. Created by Dr. Peter Levine, SE is a therapy that focuses on the body and aims to release stored trauma and restore balance to the nervous system. SE involves closely monitoring physical sensations and gently assisting the client in releasing the energy linked to past traumatic experiences.

Here's how you can practice: Locate a serene and cozy area to either sit or recline.
Take a moment to close your eyes and focus on your breath, allowing yourself to find a sense of calm and centering.
Pay close attention to your body and become aware of any areas that may be experiencing tension, discomfort, or numbness.
Take a gentle approach and direct your attention to one of these areas, simply noticing the sensations without any judgment.
Encourage the natural shifting of sensations, without imposing any changes.
When emotions or memories come up, it's important to acknowledge them and then gently redirect your attention back to your bodily sensations.
Continue this process, allowing the body to naturally release the stored energy at its own pace.
Practices to Enhance Body Awareness: Developing a heightened sense of bodily sensations can assist individuals

in recognizing and alleviating tension associated with trauma. Techniques like body scan meditation and focusing on the "felt sense" can be highly beneficial in improving body awareness.

Guided Meditation for Body Awareness:
Find a comfortable position in a calm environment.
Take a moment to close your eyes and focus on your breath, allowing yourself to relax.
Begin by directing your focus to your toes and gradually work your way up, paying close attention to any feelings of tension, discomfort, or relaxation that you may experience in your body.
Take a few moments to focus on each area of your body, simply noticing the sensations without attempting to alter them.
When you come across areas of tension, take a moment to focus on your breath and visualize letting go of the tension with each exhale.
Keep scanning until you reach the top of your head.
Emphasizing the "Felt Sense":

Find a cozy spot and gently shut your eyes.
Take a moment to focus and find your center.

Focus your attention on a specific area of your body that may be experiencing tension or discomfort.

Take note of the sensations and describe them in terms of their physical characteristics.

Embrace the sensation, accepting it without any negative thoughts or pushback.

Take a moment to consider any new understandings or changes in how you perceive the tension or discomfort.

Discover the power of breathwork techniques in regulating the autonomic nervous system, reducing stress, and promoting relaxation. These valuable tools can aid in trauma healing.

Diaphragmatic Breathing Technique:
Find a comfortable position, either sitting or lying down.

Position one hand on your chest while placing the other on your abdomen.

Breathe in deeply through your nose, allowing your abdomen to rise while keeping your chest relatively still.

Breathe out slowly through your mouth or nose, noticing your abdomen sinking.

Continue the exercise for a few minutes, paying attention to the movement of your abdomen as it expands and contracts.

Box Breathing technique:
Assume a relaxed posture with proper spinal alignment.

Breathe in slowly through your nose for a count of four.

Take a deep breath and hold it for a count of four.

Breathe out slowly through your mouth for a count of four.

Take a deep breath and hold it for a count of four.

Continue the cycle for a few minutes.

Try practicing alternate nostril breathing:

Find a comfortable seated position with good posture.

Place your right thumb over your right nostril and take a deep breath in through your left nostril.

Use your ring finger to close your left nostril, then release
your thumb and exhale through your right nostril.
Breathe in through your right nostril, then use your thumb
to close it.
Let go of your ring finger and breathe out through your left
nostril.
Keep switching between nostrils for a few minutes,
concentrating on your breathing.

Expert in Movement Therapy: Participating in mindful
movement can facilitate the release of stored trauma,
enhance body awareness, and foster emotional and physical
healing. Various forms of movement therapies, including
yoga, Tai Chi, Qigong, and dance/movement therapy, have
shown great effectiveness in promoting trauma healing.

Yoga:
Locate a peaceful area where you can engage in your
practice without any disturbances.
Start by dedicating a few moments to deep breathing,
allowing yourself to find a sense of calm and focus.
Engage in a sequence of soothing poses, directing your
attention to your breath and the physical sensations you
experience.
Include poses that encourage a sense of calm and stability,
like Child's Pose, Cat-Cow, and Legs-Up-The-Wall.
Conclude your practice by dedicating a few moments to
Savasana (Corpse Pose) for complete relaxation and to
fully absorb the positive effects.
Tai Chi is a gentle and flowing form of exercise that can
provide numerous benefits for both the body and mind. Its
slow and deliberate movements help to improve balance,
flexibility, and strength. Additionally, Tai Chi can help to
reduce stress and promote relaxation. Regular practice of
Tai Chi can be a wonderful way to enhance overall well

Locate a serene environment where you can engage in your practice without any disturbances.
Start by dedicating a few moments to deep breathing, allowing yourself to find inner balance.
Discover the art of Tai Chi by following the guidance of a knowledgeable instructor or instructional video.
Take your time as you go through the sequence, paying close attention to each movement and your breathing.
Make sure to maintain a consistent practice schedule in order to fully reap the rewards of Tai Chi over time.

Qigong:
Locate a calm environment where you can engage in your practice without any disturbances.
Start by dedicating a few moments to deep breathing, allowing yourself to find a sense of inner calm and focus.
Discover the fundamentals of Qigong by following the guidance of a knowledgeable instructor or instructional video.
Take your time and be fully present as you go through the sequence, paying attention to your breath and the way your body feels.
Consistency is key when it comes to reaping the rewards of Qigong.

Exploring the Benefits of Dance/Movement Therapy:
Locate a suitable area where you can have ample room to move around without any disturbances.
Choose music that speaks to you and motivates you to get moving.
Embrace the natural flow of your body as it responds to the music, paying attention to the feelings and emotions that emerge.
Release any preconceived notions or assumptions about your movements and savor the experience.
Take a moment to consider your emotions and any valuable

realizations that may have come to light during your workout.

Practicing mindfulness and meditation: Practicing mindfulness and meditation involves directing your attention to the present moment without passing judgment. These practices can assist individuals in cultivating a feeling of safety and empowerment, which is essential for the healing of trauma.

Practicing Mindfulness Meditation:
Discover a serene and cozy spot to sit or recline.
Take a moment to close your eyes and focus on your breath.
Direct your focus towards your breath, being mindful of the feeling of the air flowing in and out of your body.
If you find your thoughts drifting towards past trauma or distressing experiences, gently redirect your attention to your breath.
Keep going for a few minutes, gradually extending the time as you get more at ease with the routine.

Practicing Loving-Kindness Meditation:
Find a comfortable position and gently close your eyes.
Take a moment to breathe deeply and find a sense of relaxation.
Quietly recite affirmations like "May I experience safety, may I enjoy good health, may I be free from pain."
Spread these well-wishes to others by repeating phrases like "May you stay safe, may you enjoy good health, may you be free from suffering."
Keep going for a few minutes, directing your attention towards the emotions of compassion and kindness.
Guided Imagery:
Locate a serene and cozy spot to either sit or recline.
Take a moment to close your eyes and focus on your

breath.

Visualize a serene and tranquil setting, like a beach, forest, or mountain.

Engage all of your senses to create a vivid scene, immersing yourself in the sights, sounds, smells, and sensations.

Take a moment to immerse yourself in the scene, allowing your mind to unwind and savor the moment.

Incorporating Somatic Practices into Your Everyday

Routine

Incorporating somatic practices into daily routines can assist individuals in effectively managing trauma symptoms and fostering overall healing and well-being. Here are some practical tips for seamlessly integrating these practices into your daily routine:

My Morning Routine:

Begin your day by dedicating a few minutes to diaphragmatic breathing, allowing yourself to find inner balance and tranquility.

Experience the rejuvenating effects of a brief yoga or Tai Chi session to invigorate your body and mind.

Take a midday break:

Spend a few moments engaging in a body scan or focusing technique to help you identify and release any tension you may be experiencing.

Take a few moments to engage in mindful breathing or guided imagery exercises to help alleviate stress and distress associated with trauma.

Evening Routine:

Try incorporating progressive muscle relaxation or a body scan into your routine to help you unwind from the day and prepare for a restful sleep.

Try incorporating a visualization technique into your

bedtime routine to enhance relaxation and cultivate a peaceful state of mind.

During the course of the day:
Integrate mindful moments into your routine, like deep breathing, self-massage, or spontaneous movement, to effectively address trauma symptoms as they occur. Utilize grounding techniques when faced with stressful situations to maintain a sense of presence and tranquility.

The Importance of Professional Support

Although somatic practices can be highly advantageous for trauma healing, it is crucial to acknowledge the importance of seeking professional assistance. Collaborating with a knowledgeable professional in somatic therapy can offer valuable guidance, support, and a secure environment to delve into and let go of past traumas. Experts in the field of somatic therapy are skilled in assisting individuals in navigating the intricate emotions and physical sensations that often accompany trauma. They have the ability to customize interventions to suit each person's unique requirements.

When looking for professional assistance, keep the following in mind:

Qualifications and Experience: Seek out a therapist who has received specialized training and has extensive experience in somatic therapies, trauma-informed care, and possesses a profound understanding of the intricate relationship between the mind and body.

Various therapists may utilize different somatic approaches, including Somatic Experiencing, Sensorimotor Psychotherapy, or other body-oriented techniques. It's important to have a clear understanding of the therapist's approach and how it fits with your specific needs and preferences.

Establishing a solid foundation for healing trauma involves

building a strong therapeutic relationship that prioritizes safety and trust. Finding a therapist who makes you feel comfortable and supported is crucial.

Comprehensive Healing: It can be beneficial to combine somatic therapy with other forms of care, like talk therapy, medical treatment, and self-care practices, to promote holistic well-being.

Healing trauma through somatic practices provides a comprehensive and integrated approach that acknowledges the connection between the mind and body. Through a mindful approach that emphasizes bodily sensations, breath, movement, and mindfulness, somatic practices have the ability to release stored trauma, promote a feeling of safety, and enhance resilience. Various techniques, including Somatic Experiencing, body awareness practices, breathwork, movement therapy, and mindfulness, can be highly effective in promoting trauma healing.

Incorporating these practices into your daily routines can maximize their effectiveness and contribute to your overall well-being. In addition, consulting with a professional who specializes in somatic therapy can offer valuable guidance and establish a secure environment for the healing process. Whether utilized alone or in conjunction, somatic approaches provide a caring and efficient route to healing trauma and regaining a sense of completeness.

Chapter Seven

Everyday Somatic Practices for Well-being

Integrating somatic practices into your daily routine can greatly improve your overall well-being, supporting your physical, emotional, and mental health. These practices emphasize the connection between the mind and body, with a focus on awareness, movement, breath, and mindfulness. Through the incorporation of somatic practices into daily activities, individuals have the opportunity to develop a feeling of equilibrium, strength, and energy.

Exploring Somatic Practices

Somatic practices emphasize the strong connection between the body and mind. These practices emphasize the importance of being mindful of bodily sensations and using this awareness to promote overall well-being. Important elements of somatic practices include:

Developing a heightened sense of body awareness can greatly improve self-awareness and help identify any areas of tension or discomfort within the body.

Embrace the power of intentional and mindful movement to

enhance your overall well-being, both physically and
emotionally.

Discover the power of breathwork, a practice that harnesses
the potential of controlled breathing techniques to promote
a balanced nervous system and enhance your overall sense
of well-being.

Embrace the power of mindfulness to cultivate present-
moment awareness, reduce stress, and enhance emotional
resilience.

Discover the power of incorporating somatic practices into
your everyday life.

Start your day off right with a refreshing morning routine.
Beginning the day with somatic practices can create a
positive atmosphere, boost energy levels, and ready the
mind and body for the day ahead.

Start your day by dedicating a few minutes to
diaphragmatic breathing. This practice will help you find
your center and induce a sense of relaxation.

Here's a simple way to practice: Find a comfortable
position, either sitting or lying down.
Position one hand on your chest and the other on your
abdomen.

Breathe deeply through your nose, allowing your abdomen to expand while keeping your chest steady.

Breathe out slowly through your mouth or nose, noticing your abdomen sinking.

Continue the exercise for a few minutes, keeping your attention on the expansion and contraction of your abdomen.

Consider incorporating gentle stretching or yoga into your routine. Experience the rejuvenating effects of a brief session of gentle stretching or yoga to invigorate your body and mind.

Here's how to practice: Locate a calm area where you have ample room to move around.

Start by dedicating a few moments to deep breathing, allowing yourself to find a sense of calm and focus.

Engage in a sequence of soothing poses, like Cat-Cow, Child's Pose, and Downward Dog, while paying close attention to your breath and the physical sensations you experience.

Conclude your practice by dedicating a few minutes to Savasana (Corpse Pose) in order to completely unwind and incorporate the advantages.

Discover the power of incorporating mindful movement

into your morning routine. By doing so, you can enhance your body awareness and cultivate a sense of calm.

When practicing, pay close attention to the sensations in your body as you go about your morning activities. Be mindful of your body's sensations while you exercise, being aware of any areas of tightness or relaxation. Take your time and focus on each movement, fully immersing yourself in the experience.

Take a midday break

Engaging in somatic practices during the day can provide a much-needed break, reduce stress levels, boost focus, and promote overall well-being. Try incorporating a body scan meditation into your routine to help identify and release any tension you may be holding in your body.

Here's how to practice: Locate a peaceful spot to sit or lie down. Take a moment to close your eyes and focus on your breath. Begin by directing your focus towards your toes and gradually work your way up, paying close attention to any feelings of tension, discomfort, or relaxation that you may experience in your body.

Take a few moments to focus on each area of your body, simply noticing the sensations without attempting to alter them.

When you come across areas of tension, try taking deep breaths and visualizing the tension melting away with every exhale.

Keep scanning until you reach the top of your head.

Discover the power of controlled breathing techniques to bring tranquility to your mind and body.

Box Breathing: Find a cozy spot and sit with good posture. Breathe in slowly through your nose for a count of four. Take a deep breath and hold it for a count of four. Breathe out slowly through your mouth, counting to four. Take a deep breath and hold it for a count of four. Continue the cycle for a few minutes. Experience the benefits of mindful walking by engaging in a walk that promotes body awareness and helps to reduce stress.

Here's a suggestion for practicing: Look for a peaceful location where you can take a walk without any disturbances.

Start by walking at a gentle pace, focusing on the feelings
in your feet as they touch the surface beneath you.

Pay attention to the motion of your legs, the movement of
your arms, and the cadence of your breathing.

When your mind starts to drift, gently redirect your
attention to the physical sensations of walking.

Keep up the mindful walking for a few more minutes.

Evening Ritual
Concluding your day with somatic practices can assist in
unwinding, relieving the tension accumulated throughout
the day, and setting the stage for a peaceful night's sleep.

Progressive Muscle Relaxation: Incorporate progressive
muscle relaxation into your routine to effectively release
tension and encourage a state of deep relaxation.

Here's how to practice: Locate a peaceful and cozy spot to
either sit or lie down.
Take a moment to relax and focus on your breath.
Begin by tensing each muscle group for a few seconds,
starting from your toes, and then releasing.
Progress through your body, tensing and then releasing
each muscle group one by one.
Pay close attention to the feeling of calmness as you let go
of tension in every muscle group.
Utilize guided imagery to encourage a state of relaxation
and tranquility prior to going to sleep.

Here's how to practice: Locate a serene and cozy spot to
either sit or recline.
Take a moment to close your eyes and focus on your

breath.
Visualize a serene and tranquil setting, like a beach, forest, or mountain.
Engage all of your senses to create a vivid scene, immersing yourself in the sights, sounds, smells, and sensations.
Take a moment to immerse yourself in the scene, allowing your mind to unwind and savor the moment.

Evening Yoga: Indulge in a soothing yoga session to relax and let go of the day's stress.
Here's how to practice: Locate a calm area where you have ample room to move around.
Start by dedicating a few moments to deep breathing, allowing yourself to find a sense of inner calm.
Experience a sequence of calming, rejuvenating poses like Child's Pose, Legs-Up-The-Wall, and Reclining Bound Angle Pose. Pay close attention to your breath and the physical sensations you feel.
Conclude your practice by dedicating a few minutes to Savasana, allowing yourself to completely unwind and absorb the positive effects.
Throughout the Day Integrating somatic practices into your daily routine can contribute to a sense of equilibrium, alleviate stress, and promote overall well-being.

Stay present throughout the day by taking brief moments to connect with your body and breath.

Here's a simple practice you can try: Take a moment to pause and focus on your breath. Take a few deep breaths to help center yourself.
Pay attention to any areas of tension or discomfort in your body.
Take a moment to focus on those areas, visualizing the tension melting away as you breathe out.

Rediscover the joy of engaging in your favorite activities with a heightened sense of mindfulness and attentiveness.

Learn effective grounding techniques to help you stay present and calm in stressful situations.

Here's a simple practice routine: Find a comfortable position, either standing or sitting, with your feet firmly planted on the ground.
Pay attention to the feelings of your feet touching the ground.
Let's start by taking a few deep breaths, really tuning into the sensation of your breath flowing in and out of your body.
Direct your focus towards your body, being mindful of any areas that may be experiencing tension or discomfort.
Visualize a strong connection between your feet and the ground, offering a sense of stability and support.

Learn the art of self-massage to effectively release tension and induce a state of deep relaxation.
Here's how to practice: Locate a peaceful and cozy spot to either sit or lie down.
Take a moment to soothe any areas of tension by using your hands to gently massage your neck, shoulders, and lower back.
Use a gentle touch and circular movements to help alleviate tension.
Pay close attention to the sensations in your body and take deep breaths while massaging.

Discover the power of incorporating somatic practices into your everyday routines.
By incorporating somatic practices into your daily routine, you can heighten your sense of awareness and improve your overall well-being.

Discover the power of mindful eating and how it can help you savor every bite of your meals.

Here's a suggestion for practicing: Find a calm and cozy spot to sit down and enjoy your meal.
Remember to take a few deep breaths before you start your meal.
Be mindful of the colors, textures, and smells of your food.
Take small bites and savor each mouthful, paying attention to the delicious flavors and delightful sensations.
When your mind starts to drift, gently redirect your attention to the act of eating.
Discover the power of mindful cleaning to transform mundane household tasks into moments of mindfulness and relaxation.

Here's a suggestion for practicing: Select a cleaning task, like washing dishes or sweeping the floor.
Pay close attention to the sensations you experience during the activity, like the texture of the water or the motion of the broom.
Pay attention to the sights, sounds, and smells that are connected to the task.
Take slow, deep breaths and move at a relaxed pace, fully immersing yourself in the activity.
Make the most of your commute by turning it into a time for mindfulness and relaxation.

Here's a suggestion for practicing: When you're driving, try to really tune in to the sensations of the experience. Pay attention to the feel of the steering wheel in your hands and the movement of the car.
When using public transportation, it can be helpful to pay attention to your breath and the sensations of the ride.
Take a moment to fully engage your senses and observe the

world around you.

Take a moment to inhale deeply and be fully present during your commute, embracing the experience.

Discover the numerous advantages of incorporating everyday somatic practices into your routine.

Reducing Stress: Regular somatic practices can be beneficial in reducing stress levels by encouraging relaxation and alleviating bodily tension.

Enhanced Physical Well-being: Mindful movement and breathwork can work wonders for your physical health, boosting flexibility, strength, and cardiovascular function. Mindfulness and body awareness practices can help individuals stay present and manage stress more effectively, thus enhancing emotional resilience.

Enhanced Self-Awareness: Somatic practices have the ability to enhance self-awareness by fostering a deeper connection between individuals and their bodies and emotions.

Improved Sleep: Adding somatic practices to your evening routines can help you achieve better sleep by relieving tension and inducing relaxation.

Integrating somatic practices into your daily routines can greatly improve your overall well-being, supporting your physical, emotional, and mental health. Through a focus on body awareness, mindful movement, breathwork, and mindfulness, individuals can develop a sense of balance, resilience, and vitality. Incorporating these practices into your daily routine can have a positive impact on your overall well-being. By making them a part of your morning, midday, and evening, as well as throughout the day, you can experience a reduction in stress, improved physical health, and increased emotional resilience. Through various practices like yoga, breathwork, mindfulness, and self-massage, somatic techniques provide valuable tools to improve well-being and achieve a more balanced and fulfilling life

Conclusion

integrating somatic practices into your daily routine provides a comprehensive way to improve your overall well-being by nurturing the deep connection between your mind and body. These practices emphasize the importance of being in tune with your body, moving with intention, and being present in the moment. They can have a positive impact on your physical, emotional, and mental well-being. Through the incorporation of these practices into daily routines, individuals have the opportunity to develop a greater sense of equilibrium, strength, and energy, leading to a more satisfying and peaceful existence.

Discover the Strength of Mind-Body Connection Understanding and connecting with our bodies is essential in somatic practices. Through the practice of tuning into bodily sensations, individuals can develop a more profound awareness of their physical and emotional states. Through increased awareness, individuals can better recognize and alleviate tension and discomfort, promoting a state of relaxation and overall well-being. Practicing techniques like body scan meditation and mindful movement can greatly improve your awareness of your body's signals and enable you to effectively respond to its needs.

The Importance of Mindful Movement Engaging in mindful movement practices like yoga, Tai Chi, and Qigong can greatly enhance your overall well-being. These practices emphasize the importance of intentional, focused movement, which helps improve physical flexibility, strength, and balance. They also help improve emotional resilience by offering a structured method to alleviate stress and tension. Regularly practicing mindful movement can have a positive impact on your physical health, helping to reduce stress levels and cultivate a sense of inner peace and calm.

Discover the Powerful Connection Between Mind and Body Through Breathwork

Utilizing breathwork techniques can be highly effective in regulating the nervous system and inducing a state of deep relaxation. Various techniques, including diaphragmatic breathing, box breathing, and alternate nostril breathing, can be used to promote relaxation and alleviate stress and anxiety. Through the practice of mindful breathing, individuals can cultivate a feeling of stability and grounding, which can greatly assist in navigating the various obstacles encountered in everyday life. Consistent practice of breathwork can lead to improved respiratory function, heightened mental clarity, and a greater sense of well-being.

Discover the Power of Mindfulness

Practicing mindfulness helps develop a keen sense of the present moment, which is crucial for effectively dealing with stress and strengthening emotional resilience. Practicing techniques like mindfulness meditation, loving-kindness meditation, and guided imagery can help individuals stay present and minimize the effects of stress and negative emotions. Regular practice of mindfulness can help individuals gain more control over their thoughts and emotions, resulting in enhanced mental and emotional well-being.

Incorporating Somatic Practices into Your Everyday Routine

Incorporating somatic practices into everyday activities can establish a strong basis for long-term wellness. Beginning the day with deep breathing, light stretching, or mindful movement can create a positive atmosphere and ready the mind and body for the day ahead. Incorporating activities like body scan meditation, breathwork, or mindful walking into your midday routine can be beneficial for reducing stress and enhancing focus. Incorporating relaxation techniques such as progressive muscle relaxation, guided imagery, or evening yoga into your evening routine can help promote a sense of calmness and prepare your mind and body for a peaceful night's sleep. In addition, integrating moments of mindfulness, grounding techniques, and self-massage into your daily routine can contribute to a feeling of equilibrium and overall wellness.

Discover the incredible impact of somatic practices
The profound impact of somatic practices stems from their capacity to address the intricate relationship between the mind and body. Through a mindful approach that emphasizes bodily sensations, breath, and movement, these practices aim to alleviate stored tension and trauma, foster relaxation, and improve overall well-being. Consistently participating in somatic practices can result in notable enhancements in overall physical, emotional, and mental well-being, leading to a more harmonious and satisfying life.

Creating a Customized Somatic Practice Routine
In order to fully optimize the advantages of somatic practices, it is crucial to develop a customized routine that aligns with each person's unique needs and preferences. This routine is designed to be flexible and adaptable, allowing for adjustments based on changing circumstances and goals. By incorporating various wellness activities throughout the day, you can establish a tailored routine that promotes mental and physical well-being.

Looking for Expert Assistance
Although self-guided somatic practices can be quite

beneficial, it can be even more helpful to seek the assistance of a qualified somatic therapist who can offer additional guidance and insight. Experts in the field of mind-body connection provide personalized interventions and support to help individuals navigate its complexities. Seeking guidance from a knowledgeable professional can greatly improve the impact of somatic practices and create a secure environment for delving into and resolving underlying concerns.

Embracing a Holistic Approach to Well-being
Embracing a holistic approach to well-being involves a dedication to fostering the connection between the mind and body through consistent practice and self-awareness. Through the incorporation of somatic practices into everyday routines, people can establish a solid basis for long-term well-being and contentment. By incorporating techniques such as body awareness, mindful movement, breathwork, and mindfulness, somatic practices provide valuable resources to improve overall well-being and achieve a more harmonious and satisfying lifestyle.

Ultimately, somatic practices offer a well-rounded and all-encompassing approach to overall well-being, recognizing the intricate relationship between the mind and body. Through the integration of these practices into everyday life, individuals can develop a feeling of equilibrium, strength, and energy, resulting in enhanced physical, emotional, and mental well-being. Somatic practices have a remarkable ability to promote relaxation, release tension, and enhance overall well-being, making them an integral part of a healthy and fulfilling life.